Kind Climbing

Mindfulness for Responsible Mountaineering

Table of Contents

Chapter 1. Introduction

Unveiling the joy of ascending peaks while cultivating inner peace, we bring to you, our latest Special Report: "Kind Climbing: Mindfulness for Responsible Mountaineering". Filled with a sense of adventure and passion, this comprehensive guide marries the thrill of mountaineering with the serenity of mindfulness. With every turn of a page, let your curiosity pique, and allow us to accompany you on a compassionate journey towards becoming a more responsible mountaineer. No jargon, no complexity – just the pure elation of soaking in nature's grandeur while growing emotionally and ecologically. So, tie your hiking boots and grab a cup of tea – this report is bound to invigorate your spirit, and inspire you to look upon mountains with newfound reverence. Let's begin the ascent!

Chapter 2. Introducing Kind Climbing: The Blend of Passion and Responsibility

Embracing a new era of mountaineering entails an intimate dance between thrill and responsibility. Just like in life, the sport of mountaineering is most rewarding when the participant derives not only physical but also mental, emotional, and ecologic growth. This approach is encapsulated in a term of our coinage, 'Kind Climbing.' But what is it, really, at its core?

2.1. Understanding Kind Climbing

Kind Climbing goes beyond the sheer quest for adventure. It proposes a composite mindset marrying the sportsman's audacity with the ecologist's sensibility and the monk's inner peace. It accentuates the need to understand the energy and resources given by Mother Nature and maintaining the balance she craves.

At the heart of this concept lies the belief that when we ascend mountains, we do not conquer Nature but become a more integral part of it. The mountaineer is not a conqueror, rather, a humble guest, invited to revel in the beauty around every daunting ridge and cliff, amidst swirling winds and the thunderous silence that only a snow-clad peak can offer.

2.2. The Anatomy of A Kind Climber

Kind Climbing raises a new breed of mountaineer who possesses the necessary physical skill and agility but complements it with patience, respect, and thoughtfulness. A Kind Climber is enamored by the majesty of the trails, and yet remains grounded to harness the humility that nature inherently teaches.

One of the unique characteristics of a Kind Climber is their consideration of the environment. They are committed to the principle of 'leaving no trace' upon the majesty of the mountain. Their stays are defined by the lightest possible footprints, both literally and metaphorically. Not a rock disturbed, not a twig snapped, not a silent corner offended by the raucousness of human presence. This respect for the environment brings a certain mindfulness to each step taken, each breath drawn, driving the climber to take only what is necessary and leave everything else as it was found.

A Kind Climber also pays attention to safety, both their own and others around them. They continually educate themselves on the best practices and adapts these with respect to the mountains' unique temperament. They understand that their actions can have consequences not just for themselves, but also on fellow mountaineers and the mountain itself. Their choices are always weighed for their responsibility, a sense of obligation they carry with them hand in hand with their climbing gear.

2.3. Benefits of Kind Climbing

When we're armed with a mindset marrying passion and responsibility, the benefits are manifold and far-reaching.

Firstly, Kind Climbing can significantly minimize harm to these pristine mountains. Awareness and implementation of ecologically-friendly climbing practices like waste management and respectful wildlife interaction can go a long way towards preserving these natural wonders for future generations.

Secondly, the element of mindfulness that forms a cornerstone of Kind Climbing also transforms the climbing experience from just an adrenaline rush to an exercise in self-growth and self-awareness. The climber learns to respect the pace at which their body and mind wish to move, in-sync with the rhythm of nature, and enjoy every step of the journey rather than eager to touch the summit.

Lastly, this mindful approach breeds a safer climbing environment. By prioritizing precautions, safety drills, and contingency measures, not only does the individual climber feel more secure, it also builds an ethos of shared safety within the climbing community.

2.4. Cultivating The Spirit of Kind Climbing

So, how does one begin on the journey of becoming a Kind Climber? The journey may seem hard, but a few simple exercises of responsibility and mindfulness can soon habituate one into the requisite mindset.

Whether it's by meditating for ten minutes before starting the day's climb or following the principles of 'Leave No Trace,' being mindful of fellow climbers and adopting a humble attitude towards the might and sanctity of the mountain, the spirit of Kind Climbing can be cultivated with consistency and sincerity.

2.5. Conclusion

The journey to becoming a Kind Climber, like most good things in life, is gradual. But the moment you decide to trade brute force and domination for empathy, understanding, and responsibility, you've already taken your first strides toward becoming a Kind Climber. It's not just about reaching the pinnacle, but about the journey you undertake, and how that journey changes you - as an individual and as a part of this Mother Nature we all share. Despite the challenges and the harsh conditions, it's our duty to ensure that the mountain we climb is left unmolested, standing tall for generations to enjoy.

This way, we can make sure that every mountain-top experience is just as spectacular for the future adventurers as it was for us.

So, we encourage you to imbue your climbing spirit with this: Have fun, yes! But remember, to respect. To be mindful. To be kind. And then, truly, the mountains will be yours.

Chapter 3. The Pillars of Mindfulness: Applying Ancient Wisdom to Modern Mountaineering

We kickstart our journey with one of the profound truths of human existence - mindfulness, the time-tested wisdom that connects us deeply with ourselves and the world around us. Starting from the first step of the climb till the triumphant cresting of the peak, mindful presence elevates every moment of the mountaineering experience. But how can this ancient lore be attuned to the modern sport of mountaineering? A blend of two seemingly different worlds, the underlying principles remain the same. This sows the seeds for the concept of Mindful Mountaineering, a holistic approach to know not only the mountains externally but internally as well.

3.1. The Fundamentals of Mindfulness

To understand how mindfulness is applied to mountaineering, we first need to grasp its inherent essence. Mindfulness revolves around a simple yet powerful axiom: to be intensely aware of what you're sensing and feeling at every moment, without interpretation or judgment. Engaging with your senses, it's a bridge connecting you to your environment, engendering a vibrant immediacy, a direct, raw interaction with the world.

In the context of mountaineering, mindfulness encourages you to observe the world slowly opening up beneath your feet, the rhythmic crunching of your boots against the rock, the feeling of cool wind against your skin, the distant song of the birds, or your beating heart matching the intensity of the climb. The mountain becomes not an adversary to conquer, but a partner to dance with, both leading and being led, pushing and being pushed.

3.2. Moving into Mindfulness: The Practice

Mindfulness is a skill, a gently acquired capability in a distraction-filled world. The crucial step towards achieving this lies in refining one's attention. Like a lamplight in the dark, your attention helps you navigate the course of your inner terrain.

This practice begins by cultivating samatha, or calm abiding, which tethers the mind to a single point of focus. Start by focusing on your breathing – observing the sensations of your breath flowing in and out, deeply and naturally. As the mind wanders, patiently bring it back. Over time, your attention will strengthen, and distractions will cease to pull you away. You'll be completely alive, awake to this very moment.

For mountaineers, mindfulness training on breathing can also aid in altitude acclimatization. As altitude increases, air pressure drops, and breathing becomes laborious. When you convert breath into a mindfulness practice and focus on the now, it can help you deal with the physiological challenges of high-altitude hiking.

3.3. Mindful Movement: The Application in Mountaineering

The turbulence of a climb tempts one's attention to waver. However, ongoing practice will allow you to incorporate mindfulness during times of intense focus or physical hardship. This is the core of mindful movement, an application of mindfulness when in motion- focusing on the process and not on the goal, on the journey and not on the destination.

Begin by grounding yourself in the sensations of your body during the climb. Feel the pressure of your foot against the ground, the strain in your muscles, the challenging, yet satisfying, labor of your body against gravity. As you climb, your mind may start to fill with thoughts or anxieties about the future or the peak that seems increasingly elusive - here is where your practice becomes crucial. Notice these thoughts and anxieties, but gently bring your focus back to the present, to the sensation of movement, the act of climbing.

3.4. Co-existing harmoniously: Experiencing the Connection

Mindfulness is not just about you. It's an echo of your relationship with the world. As you climb, use your senses to deeply savour the richness of your environment. Respond to the symphony of sensory experiences— the rough texture of rocks, the sight of sunlight on glimmering snow caps, the rich taste of outdoor meals, the smell of fresh mountain air, and the harmony of silence.

This direct and unmediated interaction with your surroundings elevates you from being a mere visitor to someone deeply connected with the land. Every moment becomes steeped in sacredness, and mountaineering transforms into a wholesome pilgrimage, with the onus on both – reaching the pinnacle and caring for the mountains.

3.5. Compassionate Climbing: The Result of Mindful Mountaineering

Mindfulness in mountaineering, like its broader application, is ultimately about compassion. Not only do you learn to be gentle with yourself - understanding your boundaries, your strengths, your limits - but this gentleness extends to the topography you traverse.

Respect for the mountain environment becomes intrinsic, leading to conscious decisions - pitching a tent responsibly, reducing waste, being cautious not to disturb the fauna, and causing minimal environmental footprint. Mindfulness fosters a deep-seated respect for the place that hosts your journey.

In conclusion, Mindful Mountaineering gifts us the opportunity to wholly embrace the journey, transforming us into compassionate earth-keepers. As we fuse mindfulness and mountaineering, we encounter a different panorama - an intimate bond with each step we take, every height we reach, and all the challenges we overcome. Mountaineering thus becomes not just a sport of conquest, but an intimate dance of coalescence between man and mountain.

Chapter 4. Getting Equipped: Essential Gear for Conscious Climb

Mountaineering, one of the most captivating pursuits mankind has ever embarked upon, marries physical vitality with mental tenacity. But, success isn't achieved solely by physical gusto and mental courage. Equipping oneself aptly also makes a significant share of the vital prerequisites for a successful climb.

4.1. Essential Gear

Embarking on a mountaineering expedition requires careful consideration of the equipment that needs to be packed. Selecting the appropriate gear is not just about safety or comfort but also about minimizing impact on the natural environment.

Trekking Poles: Known to reduce impact on your knees, especially during descents, trekking poles are more than mere climbing accessories. They ensure stability, contributing to your overall climb's safety. Consider opting for lightweight, foldable poles designed from sustainable materials to minimize your gear's environmental footprint.

Boots and Gaiters: The importance of good quality, sturdy boots cannot be overstressed. Moreover, warmth, waterproofing, and ankle support should be considered while choosing the right pair. Gaiters, worn over the shoe and lower pant leg, are imperative to prevent snow, mud, rocks, or water from getting into your shoes.

Head Torch: A reliable, good quality head torch is essential for any climb. Opt for a torch with long battery life, and remember to pack extra batteries. Solar-powered head torches are an eco-friendly alternative helping to reduce battery waste.

4.2. Clothing for the Climb

Choosing clothing for mountaineering is a significant aspect of preparation. Base layers create the first line of defense against harsh elements, with moisture-wicking materials preventing sweat accumulation and maintaining body temperature.

Mid-layers retain body heat to protect you from cold temperatures, and down or synthetic insulated jackets are ideal choices. The shell or outer layer should be windproof, waterproof, and breathable. This includes the climbing jacket and trousers.

Gloves and mittens are necessary to protect your hands from the cold and minor injuries. Regular climbers should consider using a modular system where a thin liner is worn under heavier, waterproof gloves.

4.3. Backpack Selection

Picking the right backpack for your climb can make a world of difference. For smaller loads and shorter climbs, a 20-30 litre pack should suffice. For larger loads and long expeditions, consider a 70-90 litre backpack. Look for bags constructed from durable, lightweight materials to reduce carry weight. Also, check for adequate pocket configuration and attachment points for carrying tools and gear externally.

4.4. Climbing Hardware

Ropes, carabiners, belay devices, ice screws, and protection devices form the critical part of any climber's kit. These should comply with International Climbing and Mountaineering Federation (UIAA) safety standards. They should be lightweight and made to last, reducing both physical strain and environmental waste.

4.5. Navigation and Communication

On a climb, a reliable means of navigation can significantly improve safety and efficiency. Traditional tools such as maps and compasses can be enhanced with digital tools like GPS devices. Additionally, providing for effective communication in case of emergencies is essential. Satellite phones and personal locator beacons can be invaluable.

To conclude, becoming a conscious climber requires meticulous equipment planning and understanding the environmental impact of your gear choices. Incorporating sustainability into your mountaineering practice is just as important as getting fitted with the right gear. The planet is our playground, so taking efforts to reduce our environmental footprint will ensure that it remains pristine and beautiful for generations of thrill-seekers to come. Therefore, in the pursuits of reaching new heights, let us not forget the significant responsibility that comes with the adventure.

Chapter 5. Emotional Preparedness: Building Courage and Inner Peace

A journey into the wilderness isn't solely about the physical trek—it also requires a deep dive into the depths of your mind to plant the seeds of courage and cultivate inner peace. As a mountaineer, emotional preparedness is just as important as physical preparedness, perhaps even more. It's the amalgamation of courage, resilience, determination, and tranquility that shapes a well-rounded mountaineer.

5.1. The Importance of Emotional Preparedness

We often underestimate the power of emotional preparedness when it comes to outdoor activities, focusing predominantly on building physical strength and endurance. However, mountaineering, at its core, is as much of an emotional journey as a physical one. Being emotionally prepared equips you to handle the unexpected, remain calm under pressure, and derive enjoyment from the journey despite potential struggles. It makes the difference between feeling overwhelmed or feeling in control when faced with a challenging pass or a change in weather.

5.2. Cultivating Courage

Culturing courage is paramount when you decide to pit yourself against the might of mountains. It is not about the absence of fear; instead, it's the ability to proceed in spite of it. One can't possibly anticipate all the issues encountered in the mountains—but a prepared mind surely can tackle it better.

1. **Understanding Fear:** First, understand that fear is normal and necessary. It is your body's natural response towards potential threats, coated by a primal instinct to protect you. Recognize it, appreciate its purpose, but don't let it control your actions.

2. **Facing Fear:** Start addressing your fears by gradually exposing yourself to them. Whether it's acrophobia or nyctophobia, the key lies in slowly desensitizing your fear response until you can control it rather than it controlling you.

3. **Mental Conditioning:** Condition your mind to accept setbacks as stepping stones. Courage isn't about not failing; it's about getting back up every time you fall. A well-conditioned mind can pivot from feelings of discouragement to viewing challenges as opportunities for learning and growth.

5.3. Building Inner Peace

Just as the endless sky overlooks the mighty mountains in tranquility, your mind must learn to dwell amidst potential turmoil with calmness. Inner peace enhances your patience, clarity, and decision-making abilities; it's the silence amidst the storm.

1. **Slow Down:** Take time to slow down amidst your vigorous training regimes. Allow your mind to rest. Spend time in nature, meditate, or practice yoga—indulge in any activity that helps you connect with your inner self.

2. **Accept. Adapt. Act:** When faced with adversity, first, accept the situation. Then, adapt to what you've been given—identify your resources and acknowledge your constraints. Finally, act upon it. This sequence of actions facilitates a smoother transition through changes, fostering peace.

3. **Practicing Mindfulness:** Be present. Be aware. Whether it's the feeling of the wind against your skin or the sound of your steady

breath, observing the minutiae brings a sense of peace that refines your experiences.

5.4. Embracing Change and Uncertainty

Mountaineering promises one thing for sure—uncertainty. Weather transitions, route changes, health issues—the chronicle of a mountaineer thrives on unpredictability. Embrace it. View it as the mountain's way of telling you her untold stories.

Ways to embrace uncertainty include:

- Practising adaptability exercises.

- Visualizing different scenarios and thinking about potential responses.

- Discussing past situations where you managed change successfully.

5.5. Foster Resilience

A journey toward the peak often simulates a roller-coaster ride—with inevitable highs and lows. The resilience to withstand these ups and downs determines the color of your experiences.

- **Reframe your Perspective:** Shift your focus from the problem to the solution. Reframe your experiences not as failures, but as opportunities to learn and grow.

- **Practice Patience:** Nurture your capacity to endure difficult times without complaining. With patience, you can turn your stretches of waiting into reflective pauses essential for mental rejuvenation.

- **Practice Emotional Awareness:** Understand your emotional patterns. Awareness of when, how, and why you experience certain emotions is the first step towards mastering them.

Navigating through fears, cultivating inner peace, embracing uncertainty, and fostering resilience leads to a rewarding journey that promises more than just an ascent towards a peak. It's an opportunity to conquer the mountains within—an ascent towards a greater understanding of ourselves. Remember, it's not the mountain we conquer but ourselves.

Chapter 6. Harmony with Nature: Leaving No Trace Behind

As our forerunners began the practice of mountaineering, they left an unwritten rule for us to follow – leave no trace. This mantra, a cornerstone of responsible mountaineering, set forth the notion that we are at the behest of the beautiful, yet fragile environments we visit. Every step we take, every turn we make, we have a chance to support or disrupt this ecosystem. It's an opportunity to contribute to the longevity of these natural wonders responsibly. Let us explore how we can cultivate inner peace by honoring our immersive encounters with nature without leaving a detrimental impact.

6.1. The High Stakes

Perhaps to truly understand the concept of leaving no trace, it's important to first acknowledge the stakes. The magnificent, towering terrains that we admire so much are part of a precarious ecosystem. Flora and fauna survive in harmony, adapting to extreme weather conditions, limited resources, and isolated environments. When we set foot on a trail, it's like entering their home unannounced. They can't move their habitats, they can't protest, and they can't repair the damage we might unknowingly inflict. Therefore, it is incumbent upon us to ensure we leave no trace – an obligation that helps maintain the ecosystem's delicate equilibrium – for the integrity of their homes and our future ventures.

6.2. Start At Home: Sustainable Planning

Leaving no trace isn't just about your actions on the trail; it begins with your planning at home. By packing wisely and preparing for the trip, we can minimize the impact we make. Plan your meals to avoid packaging waste. Opt for reusable containers and utensils over disposables. Invest in high-quality gears that last longer, thus reducing the frequency of replacement and waste generation. Choose digital maps and guides over printed versions; they're not only environmentally friendly but more efficient. Most importantly, educate yourself about the specific regulations and delicate ecosystems of the area you're heading to. Familiarize yourself with local flora and fauna, potential hazards, and best practices for minimum impact camping. Knowledge is the key to responsible action.

6.3. On The Trail: Respect Boundaries

Nature thrives when we respect the boundaries. Stick to the established trails to prevent trampling sensitive vegetation. Avoid disturbing animals or interrupting their natural behaviors. Never feed them human food, as it may cause health problems and unnatural behavior changes. Resist the temptation to pick flowers or remove rocks. These might seem like small tokens, but they play a crucial role in the delicate mountain ecosystems. Leave what you find and respect wildlife – they are two of the seven principles of Leave No Trace policy.

6.4. Campsite Selection and Management

Making responsible camping choices is another crucial part of leaving no trace. Stick to established campsites and keep them small to minimize your impact. Practice 'good housekeeping' by keep your site free of food and waste, which can attract wildlife. Dispose of waste properly – pack out all trash, leftover food, and litter. If no latrines exist and you must resort to natural means, bury human waste in catholes, dug 6-8 inches deep and at least 200 feet away from water, campsites, and trails.

6.5. Fires: Think Before You Ignite

Fires have long been part of camping culture, providing both physical warmth and a communal ambiance. However, they can have an adversely lasting impact on the environment. Opt for a light-weight camp stove for cooking and a headlamp or flashlight for light. If you must have a fire, use established fire rings, keep fires small, and burn only small sticks from the ground that can be broken by hand. Always put out the fire completely and scatter cool ashes.

Innovation with minimalism and restraint is the essence of no-trace camping. The mutual respect between us as climbers and the mountains we ascend is a unique and rewarding relationship. In order to respect this connection, it's essential to practice sublime care in every action we take as we explore these majestic heights. Enacting this discipline of mindful mountaineering allows us to actively participate in nature's preservation, ensuring that these landscapes remain for future generations to treasure. Remember, as mountaineers and nature enthusiasts, we are not merely visitors but stewards of our environment. Our legacy is not how we conquer these spaces but how we respect, care, and preserve them for the future.

Chapter 7. Mental Training: Harnessing the Mind for a Smooth Ascent

Mountaineering is an arduous but rewarding endeavour. The challenges you face physically are matched only by those that test your mental fortitude. Train your mind, and you train the most essential tool you carry with you on your climbing journey. This chapter will guide you through various mental training techniques, resulting in a more serene, mindful climb, and a smoother overall ascent. Through this mental conditioning, you will see an evolution not just as a mountaineer, but also as an individual mindful of his or her place in the grand ecosystem of life.

7.1. Neuroplasticity: The Adaptable Mind

As climbers, we face adversity constantly. It's a part of the journey, and to adapt is to survive. Neuroplasticity refers to the mind's ability to alter its structure and function in response to experiences, even into old age. This mental flexibility is what allows us to learn and adapt, making us more resilient when faced with challenges.

Practice mental exercises that foster neuroplasticity such as engaging in new learning experiences, regular physical fitness, and adopting meditation. The human mind, much like a mountain, has untouched regions waiting to be explored. Unleashing your mind's potential will equip you for demanding ascents successfully under varied and unexpected situations.

7.2. Visualisation: Clear Mind, Clear Path

Visualisation is a tool used by athletes and adventurers worldwide to prepare for their next feat. This simple practice involves imagining the entire journey – from the easy walk to the hardest climb, even the summiting moment itself. See yourself overcoming physical challenges, adapting to shifting weather, and making responsible eco-friendly choices.

By immersing your mind into this visual reality, fear and anxiety can be significantly reduced. Additionally, it helps in conditioning your mind to think proactively, plan, and troubleshoot problems even before they arise. Regular visualisation will lead to a smoother, more enjoyable journey up the mountain.

7.3. Mind-Body Connection: Synching with the Self

The mind and the body are intertwined. In the high peaks, amidst cold winds and tough terrain, your body will tire. Your mind, however, can serve to keep pushing your physical boundaries, asserting control over fatigue and discomfort. The mind-body connection is the key to broadening your potential to overcome adversity.

To build a robust mind-body connection, include yoga and breathing exercises in your fitness regime. Yoga promotes flexibility, mindfulness, and balance, while breathing exercises help control heart rate and reduce fear or stress. By combining physical conditioning and mental training, you become more present, more in-sync with your body, improving your adaptability during the climb.

7.4. Mindfulness on the Trail: Preserving Inner Calm Amidst Outer Turbulence

Mindfulness on the trail is about maintaining psychological equilibrium amidst physical and environmental challenges. It involves being fully present – observing the mountain, the trail, and most importantly, the self in detail. By doing so, you learn a lot about your own behaviour, state of mind, and even discover personal metaphors that relate to life off the mountain.

Meditation sessions focusing on mindfulness, even short ones, will help you still your mind amidst the chaos. Listen as the wind rustles the leaves, feel the firm earth beneath your feet – immerse yourself fully into the serenity of nature. These peaceful moments will fuel your inner calm amidst the outer turbulence, and this tranquility will be your constant companion through the expedition.

7.5. Emotional Resilience: Cultivating Strength from Within

Climbing tests you, teases out your insecurities, your fears, yet simultaneously, it builds you. It cultivates emotional resilience, an inner strength that grows with every challenge met and every obstacle overcome.

To build emotional resilience, practice self-reflection after each climb – analyze your thoughts, your reactions, the decisions you made. This self-awareness will give you insights into your emotional health and show you areas that you can strengthen for future climbs. Over time, you will notice a stronger, more resilient version of yourself – a victor not just over the mountains, but over your own inner turmoil.

In summary, harnessing the mind is not simply about a smoother climb. It's about the journey inward while moving upward. This mental training prepares you for the physical challenges; allowing you to be proactive, remain calm, be emotionally tough, and foster a deep sense of connection with your surroundings. As your mind becomes your ally on these excursions, you also foster a sense of responsibility towards the mountains that challenge and change you. With mindfulness, every journey leaves you better – a little stronger, a little calmer, a little more at peace. So harness your mind, and let the smooth ascent begin!

Chapter 8. Sowing Respect: Understanding Mountain Cultures and Local Communities

Our journey to becoming responsible mountaineers must start with a foundation built on respect - a key attribute of mindfulness. As such, it is crucial to fully understand the realm we step into whenever we venture into the mountains. These magnificent landforms are not just landscape features; they are often intertwined with the distinctive cultures and everyday lives of the local communities. This chapter goes in-depth into the dimensions of recognizing and respecting these cultures that thrive on heights, and how to harmoniously coexist while venturing into these remarkable terrains.

8.1. High-Elevation Ethos

In many parts of the world, mountains are regarded as sacred places. For centuries, they have been viewed as the abode of deities, or the gateways to a transcendent realm. The Sherpas in Nepal consider Sagarmatha (Mount Everest) as the mother goddess of the world. Similarly, the Quechua and Aymara people hold a deep spiritual reverence for the Andean peaks which they call Apus. These perspectives influence the way locals conduct themselves in these spaces.

When you step onto such revered ground as a mountaineer, it's important to approach with a similar sense of respect. Quietly observe the rituals, gestures, and nuances in the everyday life of locals. Refrain from actions that might disrupt or upset the spiritual energy many locals believe is contained within these mountains.

8.2. Upon Their Shoulders: The Role of Mountain Communities in Mountaineering

Mountain communities play a significant role in mountaineering journeys. From guides and porters to kitchen staff and those maintaining accommodations, locals are the backbone of your adventure. They ensure your safety, direct your paths, cook your meals, and create a hospitable environment in often harsh conditions.

Understanding their roles, respecting their work, and acknowledging their expertise is a significant part of responsible mountaineering. Always remember, they are more than just service providers; they are your link to understanding the mountain and its cultural significance.

8.3. The Mountain Dialect: Language Respect and Learning

Language is an integral part of any culture, and mountain communities are no exception. Many such communities have their unique dialects, different variations of language, and specific slangs, reflecting their rich cultural history and heritage.

As an outsider, making an effort to learn a few basic phrases of the local language can work wonders in establishing rapport with the communities. It shows your respect for their culture and your willingness to be a part of it, even if only temporarily.

8.4. A Taste Of Mountain Life: Immersing In Local Customs

Mountain communities often have distinctive customs and practices that have evolved over the centuries. These traditions could be related to their food, clothing, social events, religious rituals or lifestyle practices.

Experiencing these customs firsthand can greatly enhance your mountaineering journey. As a responsible mountaineer, you ought to respect these practices, participate when invited but refrain from invading their private spaces or compelling them to perform their rituals for touristic pleasure.

8.5. Respectful Footfalls: Minimizing Impact

A large part of respecting mountain cultures and communities lies in minimizing our impact on the local ecology. Issues like littering, deforestation, or using precious resources irresponsibly can disrupt the lifestyle of the locals, in addition to wrecking ecological havoc.

To practice responsible mountaineering, strive to leave no trace of your visit. Locals depend on the mountains for their livelihood and vitality. Over-exploitation of these landscapes can compromise the health of the entire community.

8.6. Reciprocating the Hospitality: Responsible Conduct

You can expect a warm and hospitable welcome in mountain communities. Even in remote locations, locals will often go out of their way to make you feel at home. In your interactions with them, reciprocate this warmth and hospitality.

Ensure you are polite, considerate and generous. When in doubt, ask. Seek permission for photography, respect their homes and personal space, and remember that you are a guest in their world.

8.7. The Economic Elevation: Supporting Local Economies

Supporting the local economy is paramount in your journey to becoming a responsible mountaineer. Choose to stay in locally run accommodations, buy from local vendors, hire local guides, and support initiatives designed to benefit these communities.

Your monetary support directly contributes to the prosperity of these regions, facilitates poverty reduction and promotes equitable economic growth.

In conclusion, understanding and respecting mountain cultures and local communities is a vital facet of responsible mountaineering. Consciously incorporating respect for these indigenous cultures in your approach can lead to a more enriching and empathetic mountaineering experience. Remember, respect is the cornerstone of co-existence. As we venture higher into these sacred landscapes, let us also elevate our understanding, compassion, and appreciation for the rich tapestry of mountain cultures and communities that share their world with us.

Chapter 9. Responsible Risk Management: Safe Climbing and Decision-Making

Mountaineering, by its very nature, involves inherent risks. But with diligent preparation, responsible decision-making, and observational mindfulness, we can significantly mitigate these inherent risks. This is the essence of Responsible Risk Management—striking the delicate balance between the thrill of the climb and the safety of all involved, including oneself, fellow climbers, and our invaluable mountain ecosystems

9.1. Understanding the Risks

Every step taken on a mountain offers a fresh perspective, a different challenge. Before setting foot on a mountain, it's crucial to understand the risks involved. This includes recognizing potential hazards, evaluating threats, and planning accordingly.

Physical Risks chiefly comprise altitude-related issues, harsh weather conditions, unstable terrains, and the potential for rockfall or avalanches. Psychological Risks, on the other hand, encompass a range of stressors from isolation, fear of the unknown, and the pressure to succeed. Furthermore, a comprehensive understanding of the Cultural Risks involved—the respect and caution owed to local regulations, customs, and sensitive ecological areas—is an absolute must.

9.2. Dealing with Altitude

The biggest challenge prevailing in mountaineering is managing High Altitude Illness (HAI), which becomes increasingly common with altitude, from Acute Mountain Sickness (AMS), High Altitude Pulmonary Edema (HAPE), to High Altitude Cerebral Edema (HACE). As climbers ascend, oxygen levels fall, causing discomfort and potential health risks.

Understanding the symptoms is crucial. AMS typically begins with headache, fatigue, disturbed sleep, and loss of appetite. It might further evolve into HAPE (difficulty in breathing, even at rest) or HACE which can cause severe headache, vomiting, lethargy, and ataxia.

To prevent HAI, it's crucial to take things slow and let our bodies acclimate. Climb high during the day, but sleep low at night. Utilize oxygen if necessary, and take medications for symptom relief under appropriate medical supervision. Equip yourself with proper training for identifying, preventing, and treating HAI.

9.3. Navigating Harsh Weather Conditions

Weather in high altitude regions is unpredictable. Sunshine can swiftly make way for a blizzard. Hence, it becomes essential to check weather reports and be prepared for unexpected changes. Familiarize yourself with common weather patterns and always have contingency plans.

Equip yourself to endure low temperatures and potential storms. Layered clothing that can regulate body temperature while keeping moisture at bay is an essential part of any mountaineer's gear. Eye protection for bright reflective surfaces and durable tents to act as makeshift shelter during harsh storms are indispensable.

9.4. Unstable Terrains and Avalanche Safety

Mountains pride themselves on their dynamic nature, filled with rocky terrains, moving glaciers, and potential for avalanches.

Educate yourself about the different types of terrains and the specific risks they present. Seek relevant training in navigating through rocky terrains, crossing crevasses, and other terrain related difficulties. Avalanche safety predominantly involves understanding the science of snow and planning your traverse carefully, constantly evaluating the slope angle, snowpack, and changes in weather.

Invest in proper equipment such as an avalanche beacon, probe, shovel, and most importantly, gain the knowledge to use them proficiently. Participating in avalanche education courses is a good way to acquire these skills.

9.5. Embracing Mindful Decision-Making

In the face of inherent risks and fluctuating external conditions, a key factor that drives safety in mountaineering is mindfulness. This isn't just about the present moment awareness but involves a future-oriented thinking, considering the implications of our decisions, anticipating problems based on cues, and actively making informed choices.

Mindful decision-making involves being keenly aware of our skill set and limitations, understanding the group's dynamics, keeping our ambitions in check, and making decisions that prioritise safety over summiting. It's crucial to cultivate the courage to turn back when conditions aren't favourable, or when the body signals that it needs rest.

9.6. Respect for Local Customs and Ecology

Responsible mountaineering is incomplete without the understanding that the mountains have a delicate balance of life. Keeping local ecology intact while passing through these regions should be of paramount concern. Stick to designated trails without disturbing flora and fauna, carry back waste, and maintaining a bare minimum footprint is crucial as a responsible mountaineer.

Similarly, respecting local customs is the cornerstone of harmonious expeditions. For regions that are home to mountain communities, it's essential to respect local traditions, customs, and rules put forth by local governing bodies. Remember, we are visitors in their land.

In conclusion, Responsible Risk Management is not about risk aversion, but it's about undertaking the right risks, thoughtfully and proactively—an inherent responsibility each of us shares as explorers of these majestic peaks. By cultivating mindfulness, adopting new skills, and fostering an attitude of reverence towards our mountainous terrains, we enrich our experiences, safeguard our lives, and extend respect to the mountains that provide us with such incredible adventures.

Chapter 10. The Power of Solitude: Embracing Quiet Moments in the Mountains

Solitude is often interpreted as the state of being alone, an uncomfortable prospect for many. But in the realm of mountains, it can manifest as an infinitely profound experience — one that fosters deep contemplative thought, clears the mind, and amplifies the present moment's serenity. The eerie silence at a mountain's crest is an acoustic canvas upon which the grand symphony of your thoughts is played.

10.1. The Solitude Spectrum: From Silence to Inner Speech

Solitude offers a spectrum of adventure that is both inward and upward; an adventure that beckons you to explore not just the untamed beauty of the mountain, but the uncharted terrains of your mind. With solitude as your ally, one gradually observes their thought process from the lens of an outsider, identifying unnecessary cognitive chatter and tranquilizing the tumult within.

On the solitary path up a mountain, each footfall serves as a metronome for your thoughts. The journey up not only tires the body but exhausts the mind of its daily rantings until there remains nothing but the purity of silence and the rhythmic echo of your heart. That's where the transformation starts — silence gives birth to inner speech, a dialogue that's sincerely introspective yet innately empathetic. It's not mere reflection, but resonance, as your thoughts oscillate between the awe of your immediate surroundings and the depth of your sense of self.

10.2. The Mountains and Their Monastic Lessons

The mountains, in their timeless wisdom, stand as ancient monastic teachers stimulating deep reflection, compelling climbers to be more present, and fostering a meditative state. As the clutter of civilization grows fainter with elevation, the weight of distractions and obligations recedes too, making room for heightened clarity and introspection.

A mountain's spine is a winding path of solitude that promotes pause, introspection, and emotional clarity. As one ventures into the quiet realm above the tree line, the air thins, and the world is a silent articulation of majesty. Here, ensconced in a blanket of solitude, one can unearth the nurturing power of still moments.

10.3. A Heightened State of Presence

Up in the mountains, cocooned in your solitude, you'll find life doesn't buzz past in a frenzy, but unfolds gently, deliberately, moment by beautiful moment. The heightened physical demands of the climb, the stark yet surreal landscape, the isolation from routine and civilization – all these factors amplify your sense of presence.

Experience lulls you into a deeply attentive state wherein mountain details otherwise missed reveal themselves. An exotic bird's call piercing the still air, a sudden burst of wildflowers against an austere stone backdrop or the sky transforming into a billion stars' canvas – each moment is a showreel of natural grandeur to be savored in awe and gratitude.

10.4. Solitude: A Tune-up for Mental Health

The solitude found on mountain slopes presents us with a respite from life's relentless rush, an opportunity to recalibrate our thought processes and release the pent-up mental strain. Alone with your thoughts, you are, paradoxically, accompanied by your best counsel. Solitude paves the way towards mindfulness, reducing stress and anxiety, while boosting creativity and problem-solving skills.

Physical challenges combined with solitude stimulate problem-solving and decision-making capabilities, often leading to 'Eureka' moments that descend with the clarity of mountain air. In the hushed whispers of the wind and the infinite expanse of landscapes, many mountaineers claim to have discovered their life's purpose or solutions to persisting problems.

Indeed, solitude does more than just quiet your mind. It forms an essential part of our mental and emotional wellbeing, guiding us gently back to an equilibrium often lost in the hustle-bustle of everyday life.

10.5. The Empathy of Earth: A Greater Understanding of Our Role in the Natural World

An extended tenure of solitude amidst the wilderness makes you intrinsically attuned to nature. Over time, you begin to perceive subtle shifts in the ecosystem – the waxing and waning of moonlight on snow, seasonal transformations, or the delicate balance between flora and fauna. This new level of awareness reinforces empathy, reminding you of your role in the Earth's grand orchestra.

Being alone allows you to appreciate Earth for what it truly is – not merely a stage for human endeavors but a living, breathing entity unto itself. With this realization, you naturally adopt a more compassionate perspective towards the environment, one that encourages sustainable choices and responsible mountaineering.

In conclusion, solitude serves as an invigorating medicine for the cluttered mind and an empathetic tonic for the soul. Seek it in the wilderness of the mountains, where every breath you take will remind you of your connection with the entire cosmos. The peace found in these quiet moments is not a retreat from life but an intense form of engagement with it. Embrace this powerful solitude not as a condition of loneliness but the birthplace of self-discovery, environmental empathy, and profound mindfulness.

Chapter 11. Final Thoughts: From a Mountaineer to a Kind Climber

Having traveled through myriad trails, overcome numerous obstacles, basked in nature's beauty, and indulged in the practice of mindfulness, we finally find ourselves at the drawing of the curtains. This journey has undoubtedly illuminated our comprehension of how mountaineering can be both a thrill and a peaceful meditation. Before we part ways, let's consolidate our knowledge and ventures into reflexive thoughts and takeaways.

11.1. Transcending the Adventure Ascent

How often do we find ourselves entranced by a frost-kissed peak thrusting skyward, seeking to reach it, oblivious of the journey itself? Mindful mountaineering advocates for an amalgamation of destination and journey. Understanding this is to recognize the tranquil joy in every heaving breath, every muscle strain, every drop of sweat — these embody the true spirit of the adventure.

The riveting crystal clear sky, the verdant foliage, the soulful chirping of birds, the whispers of wind — all organically embody the essence of mountaineering. The journey is not solely about the climax at the peak, but more about the symphony of these experiences that add richness to our adventures.

11.2. Compassionate Trailblazing

The quest for sumptuous glory should never inflict harm on the environment. Ensure the choices we make result in the least ecological deterioration. Consider packing lightweight gear, using biodegradable products, mitigating waste, and respecting wildlife.

As mountaineers, it's essential to develop a compassionate perspective, remembering that we are mere visitors traversing through numerous ecosystems. Leaving the trails better than we found them is the cornerstone of 'Kind Climbing'.

11.3. Mindfulness: Nurturing the Inner Climber

Your physical presence on the mountain is only half the story. The profound narrative of a true mountaineer lies in the sanctity of their mind, a mind that is attuned to the rhythm of creation around them.

Through mindfulness, we train our minds to immerse in the present moment wholly. This practice leads us to recognize the intricacies of nature, enhancing our gratitude for the wilderness, and increasing our sense of responsibility towards it.

Cultivate mindfulness through conscious breathing, observing your thoughts and feelings, and embracing the humbling beauty of our environment. Allow such practices to permeate your everyday life beyond mountaineering expeditions. By doing so, you begin a journey inward - a journey to becoming a 'Kind Climber'.

11.4. Kind Climber: An Embodiment of Responsibility

From a novice mountaineer starry-eyed at every peak to a Kind Climber, the transformation is indeed profound. A kind climber is someone who takes joy in every straining muscle, finds thrill in every weary step, feeds on the adrenaline, yet savors the tranquility, embarks on the adventure, yet leaves no trace behind.

A Kind Climber appreciates the fortitude of nature and respects the vulnerability of the ecosystems cradled within the mountains. Recognizing our minuscule existence in conjunction with vast, sprawling terrains enhances our reverence for mountains and our responsibility towards their conservation.

As we reach the end of this comprehensive guide, remember that an informed and mindful mountaineer evolves into a Kind Climber. As a Kind Climber, you have a world of experiences awaiting you, each presenting new challenges and greater thrills.

Climb not only for the thrill or the health benefits but also for self-awareness, emotional growth, and ecological responsibility. Strive to better not just your climbing capabilities but also your ethical standards. Aim to scale heights and foster an environment conducive for future generations to do the same.

Each mountain we climb compels us to introspect, learn, and adapt. It's cumulative of these experiences that foster the transition - from a mountaineer to a 'Kind Climber'. The journey doesn't end here. It merely begins, onto graver challenges, thrilling adventures, and a path paved with mindfulness and empathy.

May every mountain you climb bring you closer to your inner self, and may every step you take leave the wilderness unscathed. Safe travels, mountaineer, as you embark on this beautiful journey toward becoming a kind climber.